VIAGRA

Discover How Viagra Can Help You Achieve and Maintain an Erection for Sexual Activity in Order to Increase Your Confidence in the Bedroom.

Dr. Stephen J. Miller

D1444077

Table of Contents

LONGER-LASTING ERECTIONS
MORE OPTIONS WITH TREATMENT
REDUCED STRESS AND ANXIETY
CONVENIENT TREATMENT OPTION
RAPID ONSET OF ACTION

CHAPTER 7

BEST PRACTICES FOR TAKING VIAGRA TO MAXIMIZE EFFECTIVENESS
FOLLOW YOUR DOCTOR'S INSTRUCTIONS
TAKE VIAGRA ON AN EMPTY STOMACH
DON'T TAKE VIAGRA MORE THAN ONCE A DAY.
AVOID DRINKING ALCOHOL
DON'T TAKE VIAGRA IF YOU'RE TAKING CERTAIN MEDICATIONS
DON'T TAKE VIAGRA IF YOU'RE TAKING NITRATES.
DON'T TAKE VIAGRA IF YOU'RE TAKING ALPHA-BLOCKERS
DON'T TAKE VIAGRA IF YOU'RE TAKING RECREATIONAL DRUGS

CHAPTER 8

EFFECTIVE WAYS TO IMPROVE YOUR ERECTILE DYSFUNCTION WITHOUT VIAGRA
EXERCISE REGULARLY
STOP SMOKING
LOSE WEIGHT
EAT A HEALTHY DIET
REDUCE STRESS
EXPERIMENT WITH NATURAL REMEDIES
VACUUM CONSTRICTION DEVICES
TESTOSTERONE REPLACEMENT THERAPY
TALK TO YOUR DOCTOR

CHAPTER 9

CHAPTER 10

HOW TO TALK TO YOUR DOCTOR ABOUT VIAGRA FOR ERECTILE DYSFUNCTION
MAKE A LIST OF QUESTIONS
BRING A FRIEND OR PARTNER
BE HONEST ABOUT YOUR SYMPTOMS
ASK ABOUT POSSIBLE SIDE EFFECTS
TALK ABOUT OTHER TREATMENT OPTIONS
KNOW THE COST
ASK ABOUT LIFESTYLE CHANGES

CHAPTER 11

WHAT TO EXPECT WHEN TAKING VIAGRA FOR ERECTILE DYSFUNCTION

CHAPTER 12

COMMON QUESTIONS ABOUT VIAGRA AND ERECTILE DYSFUNCTION
WHAT IS VIAGRA?
HOW DOES VIAGRA FUNCTION?
HOW LONG IS VIAGRA EFFECTIVE?
ARE THERE ANY VIAGRA SIDE EFFECTS?
WHO SHOULD NOT TAKE VIAGRA?
IS VIAGRA EFFECTIVE IN TREATING ERECTILE DYSFUNCTION?

CONCLUSION

Introduction

Viagra (sildenafil) is a prescription medication used to treat erectile dysfunction (ED), which is the inability to achieve or maintain an erection sufficient for sexual activity. Viagra should only be used as your doctor tells you to because it can have serious side effects and may not be right for everyone.

Viagra works by inhibiting the enzyme phosphodiesterase-5 (PDE5), which is responsible for breaking down cyclic guanosine monophosphate (cGMP) in the smooth muscle cells lining the blood vessels in the penis. When PDE5 is blocked, the level of cGMP goes up.

This causes the smooth muscle cells to relax and more blood to flow to the penis, which can lead to an erection.

Viagra is generally well-tolerated, but it can cause side effects in some people. The most common Viagra side effects are headache, flushing, indigestion, nasal congestion, and visual changes such as changes in color perception and light sensitivity. More serious side effects of Viagra can include priapism (a prolonged and painful erection), low blood pressure, and a heart attack or stroke.

It is important to discuss the potential risks and benefits of Viagra with a healthcare provider before starting treatment. Viagra is not suitable for everyone and is not recommended for use in women or children. It is also not recommended for people who are taking nitrates or alpha-blockers, who have certain medical conditions, such as liver or kidney disease, or who have had a heart attack or stroke in the past.

Viagra is a useful treatment option for many men with ED, but it is not a cure for the condition. To effectively manage the condition, it is important to address any underlying causes of ED, such as physical or psychological conditions. A healthcare provider can assist in determining the cause of ED and recommending appropriate treatment options, including Viagra, if necessary.

Chapter 1

Symptoms of Erectile Dysfunction

Erectile dysfunction (ED) is a common male condition that affects the ability to achieve and maintain an erection. It can be caused by physical or psychological factors or a combination of both. While it is not uncommon for men to experience difficulty achieving or maintaining an erection at some point in their lives, it is important to be aware of the symptoms of erectile dysfunction so that you can seek treatment as soon as possible.

The most common symptom of erectile dysfunction is difficulty achieving or maintaining an erection. This may include the inability to get an erection or an erection that does not last long enough for satisfactory sexual activity. Other symptoms that may indicate ED include reduced sexual desire, difficulty achieving orgasm, premature ejaculation, and a lack of morning erections.

In addition to the physical symptoms, there may also be psychological symptoms associated with ED. These can include anxiety, depression, low self-esteem, and feeling ashamed or embarrassed about the condition. It is important to understand that these psychological symptoms can also contribute to ED.

ED affects millions of men each year, and the symptoms can have a wide range of variations. While some men may have difficulty achieving an erection, others may experience a sudden or gradual loss of an erection during sexual activity. Reduced interest in sex is another common symptom of ED, and physical or psychological factors can cause it.

ED can be a source of stress or anxiety, especially when it begins to affect relationships or intimacy. It can be difficult to predict whether an erection will occur or not, and this can lead to frustration and even embarrassment. It is important to seek medical help as soon as possible if you suspect you might be suffering from ED. Treatment options for ED are available, ranging from lifestyle changes to medication and surgery.

Changes in lifestyle, such as giving up smoking and becoming more physically active on a regular basis, have been shown to improve overall health and lower the risk of erectile dysfunction (ED).

Medication can be used to help with the symptoms of ED, and a variety of medications are available to treat different kinds of ED. Lastly, surgery can be an option for some men and can be effective in restoring erectile function. It is important to remember that ED is a common problem, and there is no need to be embarrassed about it. Seeking medical help is the best way to ensure that the right treatment is found. ED can profoundly affect relationships, but it is not something to be ashamed of. With the right treatment and lifestyle changes, many men can experience relief from the symptoms of ED and have happier, more fulfilling relationships.

Chapter 2

Effects of Erectile Dysfunction in Sexual Life

When it comes to erectile dysfunction, the phrase "quality of life" often comes to mind. Erectile dysfunction (ED) is the inability to achieve or maintain an erection sufficient for sexual activity. A variety of physical and psychological conditions can cause it. Unfortunately, ED can significantly impact a person's sexual life and overall quality of life.

ED can affect a person's self-esteem and confidence, and it can lead to feelings of anxiety and depression. ED can also cause intimacy and communication problems, leading to relationship issues and even breakups. Not only can the physical aspects of ED have a negative impact on one's quality of life. It can also affect the mental and emotional aspects. ED can cause stress and affect a person's ability to enjoy and participate in a sexual activity fully. It can also lead to feelings of frustration and disappointment, which can impact a person's overall happiness and satisfaction with life.

If you are experiencing ED, there are a few things you can do to help yourself. The first step is to discuss the matter with your primary care physician. They will be able to assist you in determining whether or not there is an underlying medical condition that may be causing your ED.

In addition, there are lifestyle changes you can make to help improve your ED, such as exercising regularly and eating a healthy diet. You can also seek counselling if you feel like your ED is affecting your mental health.

Finally, there are treatments available for ED. There are medications, such as Viagra, Cialis, and Levitra, that can help improve blood flow to the penis and increase a man's ability to achieve and maintain an erection. In addition, some men find that using mechanical aids such as a penis pump or penile implant can be beneficial.

ED can significantly impact a person's sexual life and overall quality of life. It can cause feelings of anxiety, depression, and frustration. It can also lead to relationship issues and breakups. Fortunately, treatments available can help improve ED and help a person maintain a fulfilling and enjoyable sex life. If you are experiencing ED, talk to your healthcare provider about the best treatment options for you.

Chapter 3

The Latest Research on Viagra and Erectile Dysfunction

When it comes to the treatment of erectile dysfunction (ED), the medication known as Viagra (sildenafil) is one of the most well-known and researched options available.

Recent studies have focused on the use of Viagra in combination with other treatments because it has been shown to be an effective treatment for erectile dysfunction (ED) in a large number of men.

One study, conducted in 2020 and published in the Journal of Sexual Medicine, investigated the efficacy of treating erectile dysfunction (ED) with a combination of Viagra and tadalafil (Cialis).

The study found that this combination was more effective in improving erectile function than either medication alone or tadalafil (Cialis) alone in treating ED. The study found that this combination was more effective in improving erectile function than either medication alone. This suggests that, for some men, a combination of two medications may be more effective than one.

Other research has looked at the use of Viagra in combination with physical therapy or behavioral therapy for ED. A study published in the Journal of Sexual Medicine in 2019 found that combining Viagra and pelvic floor muscle exercises effectively improved sexual function in men with ED. This suggests that, for some men, combining medications with other treatments, such as exercise, may be more beneficial than just taking medication alone.

While Viagra is an effective treatment for ED, it is important to remember that it is only available with a prescription and should be used under the direction of a healthcare provider. Viagra should not be taken without consulting a healthcare provider, as it can interact with other medications and cause side effects. Additionally, Viagra should not be used if someone takes nitrates for chest pain or heart problems.

Overall, Viagra is a widely studied and effective treatment for ED and can be used in combination with other treatments, such as exercise and behavioral therapy, for improved outcomes. If you are considering taking Viagra for ED, talk to your healthcare provider to determine if it is the right choice.

Chapter 4

Why Using Viagra to Treat Erectile Dysfunction

E rectile dysfunction, people also refer to as ED, is a condition that affects millions of men all over the world and causes them to have difficulty getting and keeping an erection. This condition can be quite embarrassing. Although there are many treatments available for erectile dysfunction (ED), one of the most well-known of these is Viagra. But what many people don't realize is that Viagra is not a cure for ED, and it is important to address any underlying causes of the condition, such as physical or psychological conditions.

When it comes to treating ED, a healthcare provider can help determine the cause of the condition and recommend the best treatment options for each individual. This includes lifestyle changes, medications, or a combination of both. In some cases, medications like Viagra may be recommended to help improve the symptoms of ED. However, it is important to discuss the potential risks and benefits of Viagra with a healthcare provider before starting treatment.

When taking Viagra, you run the risk of experiencing a number of side effects, such as headaches, heartburn, nasal congestion, and blurred vision, among other things. Additionally, Viagra should not be taken by men who take nitrates for chest pain, as it can cause a dangerous drop in blood pressure. It is also crucial to talk to a health provider before taking any other medications while taking Viagra.

Viagra will not cure ED, but it can help to improve the symptoms. When used correctly, Viagra can help men achieve and maintain an erection during sexual activity. However, it is important to remember that Viagra should not be used as a substitute for proper medical attention and treatment. A healthcare provider can help to determine the cause of ED and recommend the best treatment options for each individual.

Ultimately, it is important to remember that Viagra is not a cure for ED and that it is important to address any underlying causes of the condition, such as physical or psychological conditions. A healthcare provider can assist in determining the cause of ED and recommending appropriate treatment options, including Viagra, if necessary. It is important to discuss the potential risks and benefits of Viagra with a healthcare provider before starting treatment.

Chapter 5

Overcoming Performance Anxiety with Viagra for Erectile Dysfunction

Performance anxiety is one of the common causes of erectile dysfunction (ED), which is the inability to achieve or maintain an erection sufficient for sexual activity. Viagra (sildenafil) is a prescription drug used to treat ED. In some cases, it can also help people with performance anxiety.

Performance anxiety can occur when a person becomes anxious or stressed about their sexual performance, which can lead to ED. This can be a cycle, as ED can lead to further anxiety and stress, which can then lead to more ED.

Viagra works by inhibiting the enzyme phosphodiesterase-5 (PDE5), which is responsible for breaking down cyclic guanosine monophosphate (cGMP) in the smooth muscle cells lining the blood vessels in the penis. When PDE5 is blocked, the level of cGMP goes up. This causes the smooth muscle cells to relax and more blood to flow to the penis, which can lead to an erection.

Viagra is generally well-tolerated and is effective in a large number of men suffering from ED. It is taken orally, usually as a tablet, and can be taken with or without food. The effects of Viagra usually last between four and six hours, but this can depend on the person and other things, like how bad the ED is and if they have other health problems.

While Viagra can effectively overcome performance anxiety in some cases, it is not a cure for ED. It is important to address any underlying causes of the condition, such as physical or psychological conditions.

A healthcare provider can assist in determining the cause of ED and recommending appropriate treatment options, including Viagra, if necessary. It is important to discuss the potential risks and benefits of Viagra with a healthcare provider before starting treatment.

Chapter 6

Benefits of Taking Viagra for Erectile Dysfunction

Viagra is a powerful prescription medication that can help you get your sex life back on track. It is a drug that has been shown to help men with ED get and keep an erection during sexual activity.

If you're considering taking Viagra for erectile dysfunction, it's important to understand the benefits it can provide.

Below are the highlighted benefits of taking Viagra for ED:

Improved Sexual Performance

Viagra has been shown to be effective in improving sexual function in many men with ED. It can help you get and keep an erection strong enough for sexual activity, which can make you feel closer to your partner and more satisfied with sexual activity in general.

Enhanced Confidence

Taking Viagra can help men with ED feel more confident about their sexual performance. This can be especially beneficial for men who have struggled with ED for a long time.

Longer-Lasting Erections

Viagra helps men achieve and maintain an erection longer than they could without the medication. This can make sex more enjoyable for both partners.

More Options with Treatment

Viagra can be taken in pill form or injected into the penis. Different options are available, depending on what works best for each individual.

Reduced Stress and Anxiety

Viagra helps reduce stress and anxiety associated with ED. This can be especially helpful for men who experience performance anxiety regarding sex.

Convenient Treatment Option

Viagra is taken orally, usually as a tablet, and can be taken with or without food. It is a convenient treatment option for many men with ED.

Rapid Onset of Action

Viagra typically begins to work within about 30 minutes to an hour after it is taken. The effects can last for four to six hours. This can make it a useful treatment option for men needing a quick ED solution.

8. Widely available: Viagra is widely available and is widely prescribed by healthcare providers for the

treatment of ED. It is also available in generic form, which can be more affordable than the brand-name medication.

Suppose you're considering taking Viagra for ED. In that case, it's important to talk to your doctor to ensure it's the right decision.

Your physician will be able to provide you with additional information regarding the possible benefits and risks of using Viagra and other treatment methods for ED, such as making changes to your lifestyle and seeking counseling.

Viagra is an effective treatment for ED, and it can help you get your sexual life back on track. With the right approach and treatment, you can experience improved sexual performance, enhanced confidence, and longer-lasting erections. Talk to your doctor today to learn more about the potential benefits of taking Viagra for ED.

Chapter 7

Best Practices for Taking Viagra to Maximize Effectiveness

Taking Viagra is one of the most effective ways to treat erectile dysfunction. However, to maximize its effectiveness and minimize the risk of side effects, it's important to follow the recommended practices when taking Viagra. Here are some tips for maximizing the effectiveness of Viagra:

Follow Your Doctor's Instructions

Before taking Viagra, talk to your doctor about the proper dosage and any other instructions they may have. It's important to take the right amount of Viagra at the right time to maximize its effectiveness.

Take Viagra on an Empty Stomach

Viagra works best when taken on an empty stomach. Taking it with food or drinks can reduce its effectiveness.

Don't Take Viagra More Than Once A Day.

Taking Viagra more than once a day can increase the risk of side effects and reduce its effectiveness.

Avoid Drinking Alcohol

Drinking alcohol can reduce the effectiveness of Viagra. Also, drinking alcohol can increase the risk of side effects.

Don't take Viagra if you're taking certain medications

Certain medications can interact with Viagra, so it's important to talk to your doctor if you're taking any medications. This includes medications for high blood pressure, heart disease, and depression.

Don't take Viagra if you're taking nitrates.

Nitrates are used to treat chest pain. Taking Viagra with nitrates might lead to a dangerous drop in blood pressure.

Don't Take Viagra If You're Taking Alpha-Blockers

Alpha blockers are medications used to treat an enlarged prostate. Taking Viagra with alpha-blockers can cause a dangerous drop in blood pressure.

Don't Take Viagra If You're Taking Recreational Drugs

Taking recreational drugs, such as ecstasy and cocaine, can increase the risk of side effects with Viagra.

By following these tips, you can maximize the effectiveness of Viagra and minimize the risk of side effects. It's important to talk to your doctor before taking Viagra to ensure it's safe for you.

Chapter 8

Effective Ways to Improve Your Erectile Dysfunction without Viagra

Erectile dysfunction (ED) is a common problem that affects many men. It can be caused by numerous factors, including physical and psychological ones. The good news is that there are many effective ways to improve your erectile dysfunction without having to resort to taking Viagra.

Exercise regularly

Exercising regularly can help you to improve your overall health and well-being, which can in turn help to improve your erectile dysfunction.

Exercise increases blood flow and oxygen to the penis, both of which are important for achieving and maintaining an erection. Regular exercise can also help reduce stress, which can majorly cause ED.

Stop Smoking

Smoking can have a negative impact on your overall health, including your erectile function. Tobacco smoke can damage the lining of the blood vessels in the penis, leading to reduced blood flow and difficulty achieving and maintaining an erection. Quitting smoking can improve your overall health as well as your erectile function.

Lose Weight

Being overweight can have a negative impact on your erectile performance. Excess weight can reduce your testosterone levels and increase the risk of developing diabetes or high blood pressure, which can lead to erectile dysfunction. Losing weight can help reduce your risk of developing ED.

Eat a Healthy Diet

A healthy diet is an important part of overall health and can help improve your erectile function. Consuming various fruits and vegetables, lean proteins, and healthy fats can help improve your overall health and reduce your risk of developing ED.

Reduce Stress

Stress can have a negative impact on your overall health, including your erectile function. Stress can lead to difficulty achieving and maintaining an erection. Reducing your stress levels can help to improve your overall health as well as your erectile function.

Experiment with Natural Remedies

Some natural remedies can help improve your erectile function. Ginkgo biloba, horny goat weed, and other natural supplements can help to improve blood flow and circulation to the penis, making it easier to achieve and maintain an erection.

Vacuum Constriction Devices

These are made of a plastic cylinder and a pump. They achieve their effect by creating a vacuum around the penis, which encourages an increase in blood flow and ultimately results in an erection.

Testosterone Replacement Therapy

Low testosterone levels can contribute to ED, and testosterone replacement therapy can help improve sexual function in some men.

Talk To Your Doctor

If you are having difficulty achieving or maintaining an erection, you must talk to your doctor. Your doctor can help identify any underlying causes of your ED and recommend treatment options that are best for you.

Erectile dysfunction is a common problem but does not have to be permanent. There are many effective ways to improve your erectile dysfunction without having to resort to taking Viagra. It is possible to improve your erectile function by, among other things, adopting a healthier diet, quitting smoking, engaging in regular physical activity, and lowering your stress levels. If none of these solutions works, you need to make an appointment with a medical professional to receive the appropriate care.

Chapter 9

Viagra-Safe Alternatives

Viagra has been the go-to drug for treating ED for many years. Still, the potential side effects and interactions with other medications can be concerning. Fortunately, a variety of alternative treatments for ED are available that can be just as effective as Viagra but without the potential side effects. PDE-5 inhibitors are one of the most popular Viagra alternatives. These drugs can help relax the muscles in the penis, allowing more blood to flow into the penis and thus helping to achieve and maintain an erection. Common PDE-5 inhibitors include sildenafil (Viagra), tadalafil (Cialis), and vardenafil (Levitra). While these medications are generally safe, it is important to note that they can interact with certain other medications and should be discussed with your doctor. If you are looking for a natural, herbal alternative to Viagra, there are several options available. Herbal supplements are often used to treat ED, such as ginkgo biloba, horny goat weed, and Asian ginseng. These supplements can help improve blood flow to the penis, helping to achieve and maintain an erection. However, it is important to note that herbal supplements are not regulated by the FDA and should be discussed with your doctor before taking them.

Another option for treating ED is a vacuum device, which can be used to create an erection by drawing blood into the penis. This device is often recommended for men who have had difficulty achieving or maintaining an erection with other treatments.

However, it is important to talk to a doctor to ensure this device is safe for you. Finally, lifestyle changes can also help treat ED. Exercise and a healthy diet can help improve blood flow to the penis and reduce stress, which can help improve sexual function. Quitting smoking can also help improve blood flow to the penis. Overall, several Viagra alternatives are safe for your health and can help you achieve and maintain an erection.

It is critical to have a conversation with your medical provider to establish whether or not the treatment option you are considering is appropriate. Alterations to your way of life along with the appropriate medical care can put you on the path to having a sexual life that is both healthy and fulfilling.

Chapter 10

How to Talk to Your Doctor about Viagra for Erectile Dysfunction

When it comes to erectile dysfunction, Viagra is one of the most talked-about treatments. Viagra (sildenafil citrate) is a medication used to treat erectile dysfunction, a condition in which a man cannot get or maintain an erection. It relaxes the muscles in the penis and increases blood flow to the area, resulting in an erection.

Suppose you have erectile dysfunction and are considering Viagra as a treatment option. In that case, you must speak to your doctor about it. Below are some tips to help you have a productive conversation with your doctor about Viagra for erectile dysfunction.

Make a List of Questions

Before you talk to your doctor, take some time to write down any questions you may have about Viagra and erectile dysfunction. This will ensure that you don't forget to ask important questions and can help you feel more prepared for the conversation.

Bring a Friend or Partner

If it's helpful, you should bring a friend or partner to the appointment. This person can provide moral support and help you remember any questions or points you want to discuss.

Be Honest About Your Symptoms

Your doctor can only help you if you are upfront and honest about your symptoms. If you are embarrassed about the condition, don't be. This is a very common problem; your doctor will understand and not judge.

Ask About Possible Side Effects

It's important to talk to your doctor about any potential side effects you may experience with Viagra. Side effects can include headaches, flushing, and an upset stomach.

Talk about Other Treatment Options

Your doctor may suggest other treatments for erectile dysfunction. If you are uncomfortable using Viagra, discuss potential alternatives with your doctor.

Know the Cost

Be sure to ask your doctor about the cost of the medication and any additional expenses, such as copays or deductibles.

Ask About Lifestyle Changes

Your doctor may suggest lifestyle changes to help with your erectile dysfunction. These can include eating a healthy diet, exercising regularly, and avoiding activities such as smoking and drinking alcohol.

Talking to your doctor about Viagra for erectile dysfunction is important in finding the right treatment option. Use these tips to help make the conversation go as smoothly as possible.

Chapter 11

What to Expect When Taking Viagra for Erectile Dysfunction

Viagra has long been considered a go-to solution for many men. Since its launch in 1998, this drug has helped millions of men around the world overcome the symptoms of ED. But what should you expect when taking Viagra for ED?

First, it's important to remember that Viagra is a prescription drug that should only be taken after consulting with a doctor. Your doctor will be able to look at your specific needs and decide if Viagra is the best choice for you.

Once you've been prescribed Viagra, you'll need to take the pill with some form of sexual stimulation (such as touching or kissing) to take effect. Depending on your prescribed dosage, you can expect Viagra to start working within 30 minutes to an hour after taking it. When you take Viagra, its effects can last up to 4 hours. However, it's important to remember that the length of time Viagra works varies from person to person.

The most important thing to remember when taking Viagra for ED is that it is not a cure-all for the condition. It can help improve the symptoms of ED but cannot cure it. Viagra is a very safe medication, but it can cause some side effects in some people. Most people who take Viagra will get a headache, a flushed face, an upset stomach, a runny nose, or feel dizzy. If you notice these symptoms, you must speak to your doctor immediately.

Finally, it's important to remember that Viagra is not a substitute for psychological therapy or counseling. If you're suffering from ED, it's important to seek professional help to treat the underlying causes.

By following your doctor's instructions and using Viagra correctly, you can expect to start feeling positive results from the medication within the first few weeks of use. With careful use, Viagra can be an effective treatment for ED and help you to regain your sexual confidence and enjoy healthier sex life.

Chapter 12

Common Questions About Viagra and Erectile Dysfunction

E rectile dysfunction (ED) is a very common condition among men of all ages, and Viagra is one of the most popular treatments for ED. But there are still many questions about how Viagra works and what it can do for men with ED. This guide will answer some of the most common questions about Viagra and erectile dysfunction.

What is Viagra?

Viagra (sildenafil) is a prescription medication used to treat erectile dysfunction in men. It increases blood flow to the penis, allowing men to achieve and maintain an erection during sex. Viagra is available in both tablet and liquid form.

How Does Viagra Function?

Viagra works by blocking the breakdown of a chemical called cGMP, which helps relax the smooth muscle cells in the penis. This action increases blood flow to the penis, allowing men to achieve and maintain an erection. Viagra is not an aphrodisiac and will not cause an erection.

How Long Is Viagra Effective?

The effects of Viagra usually last for around four hours. However, the time that Viagra remains effective varies from person to person. Some men may experience the effects of Viagra for up to eight hours.

Are There Any Viagra Side Effects?

The most common noticeable side effects of Viagra are mild and include headaches, flushing, a stuffy nose, indigestion, and dizziness. Less common side effects can include vision changes, pain in the arm or leg, and chest pain.

Who should not take Viagra?

Viagra is not recommended for men who take nitrates for chest pain. It can also interact with certain drugs, such as alpha-blockers and certain antibiotics, so it's important to talk to your doctor before taking Viagra. If you are pregnant or breastfeeding, Viagra is not recommended.

Is Viagra Effective in Treating Erectile Dysfunction?

Viagra can help men with ED achieve and maintain an erection for successful intercourse. It is important to remember that Viagra is not a cure for ED and may not work for everyone. Your doctor can help determine if Viagra is the right treatment for you.

In conclusion, Viagra is one of the most popular treatments for erectile dysfunction. It increases blood flow to the penis, allowing men to achieve and maintain an erection. Viagra is available in tablet and liquid form, and the effects usually last around four hours. However, Viagra is not recommended for all men, so it's important to talk to your doctor before taking it.

Conclusion

Viagra (sildenafil) is a prescription medication used to treat erectile dysfunction (ED), which is the inability to achieve or maintain an erection sufficient for sexual activity. It works by inhibiting the enzyme phosphodiesterase-5 (PDE5), which is responsible for breaking down cyclic guanosine monophosphate (cGMP) in the smooth muscle cells lining the blood vessels in the penis. This leads to the relaxation of the smooth muscle cells and increased blood flow to the penis, which can result in an erection.

Viagra is generally well-tolerated and is effective in a large number of men suffering from ED. It is taken orally, usually as a tablet, and can be taken with or without food. The effects of Viagra usually last between four and six hours, but this can depend on the person and other things, like how bad the ED is and if they have other health problems.

While Viagra can be an effective treatment option for ED, it is not a cure for the condition, and it is not appropriate to use it as a long-term solution. It is important to discuss the potential risks and benefits of Viagra with a healthcare provider before starting treatment and to follow the instructions provided by the healthcare provider when taking the medication. It is also important to address any underlying causes of ED, such as physical or psychological conditions, to effectively treat the condition.